Changing Lives—

ONE SMILE AT A TIME

ERIC R. TURKE, D.D.S.

Changing Lives—
ONE SMILE AT A TIME

What Every Parent Needs to Know about Orthodontics

Advantage®

Published by Advantage, Charleston, South Carolina.
Member of Advantage Media Group.

Printed in the United States of America.

10 9 8 7 6 5 4 3 2 1

ISBN: 978-1-59932-942-0
LCCN: 2018935306

TABLE OF CONTENTS

Foreword

From the Founder of Excellence in Orthodontics

MY NAME IS DR. DUSTIN BURLESON. I'm an orthodontist and the founder of Excellence in Orthodontics. My reasons for becoming an orthodontist and forming a national organization for exceptionally successful orthodontists leading the field in both clinical and patient care—instead of becoming a veterinarian or handsome movie actor or professor of poetry—are easily found at ExcellenceinOrthodontics.org, if you're curious. They might matter to you.

But this book is about *you,* the parent, and your son or daughter, not about me. It's about information you need to know to make intelligent, responsible decisions about your child's health, appearance, self-esteem, and social interactions … of a permanent, lifelong nature. Does your child really *need* braces? If so, when? If so, who should you trust to provide his orthodontic care? How will you know you're not being ripped off?

If you take the time to read this book, you'll know how to confidently and correctly make whatever decisions you need to make about your child's orthodontic care.

To start, we're no longer dealing with heavy, ugly, tight, painful metal braces—every visit to have them tightened was another round of torture; they were hard to put on, hard to keep on, painful to remove, and it was irritating having a list of foods and activities to avoid for a long period of time. If your child needs braces now, the experience won't be anything like it was when you were a kid.

Not only has *everything* about braces changed, but now all braces are created differently. So try to get that horrible, metal-mouth image out of your head. You're probably aware of invisible braces, maybe by a brand name: Invisalign. That's what prompts a lot of patients to call or email me in the first place. However, Invisalign is but one of a number of options to be considered to get to *the* best, customized, and personalized answer to your child's needs. You don't want to equate this to buying something over the counter: "Hey, give me Invisalign. How much?" It's more complicated than that. But it's a good representation of modern braces. They can be (nearly) invisible, pliable and with lighter steel, safer, and even self-removable for hygiene or sports and easily put back in place. They're not painful and achieve more certain results in a shorter period of time.

When I was growing up, a lot of kids didn't get braces they really needed and their parents let them off the hook, either because they believed their child couldn't tolerate the pain or because the cost was just beyond the family's budget. Now, braces are virtually painless, and there are flexible payment options to meet the family budget.

"My 13 year old daughter was a patient of Dr. Turke. She had an overjet and a crossbite, but after her orthodontic treatment she now has a beautiful smile! We are so grateful to Dr. Turke!"

—FAYE T.

More Than Just Braces

My second introductory message is: this is about more than just braces.

Orthodontic care for a child, preteen, or teen is more than just correcting crooked, crowded teeth with braces. That's like thinking diabetes only needs attention when feet have to be amputated, or getting tires checked might be a good idea after being stranded with a flat at night while it's pouring rain.

Orthodontic checkups *by an orthodontist*[1], starting at age eight or nine, are a proper part of child rearing. In many cases, prevention is less troublesome and less costly. Even if you're late getting your son or daughter in, it's still possible they won't need braces and that other treatment options will do. But if they do need braces, the sooner you know of the options, the better.

This is also about more than just braces because it impacts psychological and emotional health, not just oral health. This is discussed later in the book.

Why It's Important

1. Both kids and adults with great smiles feel better about themselves, and that can greatly increase their confidence.
2. Speech is greatly enhanced once teeth are better aligned.
3. Better digestion is greatly improved due to a new bite improvement.

---

1 All orthodontists are dentists, but dentists are *not* the same as or suitable substitutes for orthodontists. Read on to find out more.

4. People with straight, well-aligned teeth can avoid gum disease, which has very serious health ramifications.

5. Properly aligned jaws may reduce the risk of temporomandibular joint disorders (TMJ), which can ruin sleep or cause chronic headaches or migraines.

6. Straight teeth function better, are easier to clean, and are more likely to last a lifetime.

Some parents put off orthodontic treatment, but these irregularities and problems do *not* heal themselves. *This isn't acne; they don't grow out of it.* The problems only grow worse and harder to resolve with age.

Don't Ask Them to Hide Their Smile

Never smiling isn't easy in an age of selfies and social media. Children can become self-conscious—painfully self-conscious—and embarrassed. "No thanks, Mom, I'd rather just stay home."

Teen suicide has skyrocketed since social media shaming and bullying rose to ugly prominence. Teen depression affects everything from getting the good grades needed to get into a good college to first dates, first loves, and enjoying (or hating) their childhood and teen years. But it doesn't stop there. Uncorrected, bad smiles go with them to college and into their career.

This isn't just cosmetic either. It's also medical and can be a serious detriment to their health.

So, read on. Be informed. Be able to ask smart questions and do the right thing. I guarantee you'll be much better able to correctly and confidently make good choices for your family through this book.

Dr. Dustin S. Burleson, DDS

Founder, Excellence in Orthodontics

Clinical Professor, The University of Missouri Kansas City School of Dentistry, Department of Graduate Orthodontics & Dentofacial Orthopedics

Adjunct Professor, The Children's Mercy Hospital, Kansas City, Missouri, Department of Cleft & Craniofacial Orthodontics

Director, The Rheam Foundation for Cleft & Craniofacial Orthodontics

Introduction

EVERYONE CONSIDERING ORTHODONTICS for themselves or their children needs to know that orthodontics does change lives. Orthodontics involves improving one's self esteem, improving dental and nutritional health and improving speech all by changing one's bite. My intent in writing this book isn't necessarily to entertain, but to inform.

Orthodontic treatment is a pretty big investment in both time and money, so I understand parents and patients want to know more about what to expect and how the whole process works. One of my goals is to give you the confidence to make right decisions concerning orthodontic treatment for yourself or your child.

In this book, you will find the most commonly asked questions about orthodontics, and questions you may have never known you have. I hope you enjoy reading this book to find out what everyone needs to know about orthodontics.

Yes, orthodontists do change lives—one smile at a time!

Chapter One

Why Is My Child's Smile So Important?

IF YOU ARE WEIGHING the yes/no and now/later decisions of orthodontic care or braces, you'll be trying to decide just how important or unimportant it really is.

Some parents feel "looks aren't everything." Some think their kid should just be tough-minded about this and not overly sensitive. Some may not have had orthodontic care when they were children and think, *Hey, I turned out just fine. I have a great spouse, a good career, friends—so what's the big deal?*

But that was then. This is *now*: the age of social media.

Social shaming and bullying is a lot worse, a lot more common, and a lot more persistent than when you were a kid. Teen suicide is on the rise, and such suicides share one thing in common: shocked and bewildered parents who could not conceive of their child ending his own life. Sure, they might've noticed he was a *little* depressed and withdrawn. They knew he was being bullied and spending more time home, alone, not leaving his room, but geez, he *is* a teenager, after all. What once was a few days or weeks of misery contained in the cafeteria with a few bullies is now endless, expansive, and broadcast online to everybody. Behind a computer screen, it can get far nastier than most would dare in person. Sometimes, kids bully each other for no reason, being a buck-toothed girl or a boy with gaps in between their teeth is enough to exacerbate the situation.

Signs Your Child May Be Being Bullied

- decrease in self-esteem
- not wanting to go to school
- skipping school
- injuries they can't explain
- self-destructive behaviors (e.g., harming themselves)
- declining school grades
- sleep difficulties
- loss of interest in schoolwork or activities
- sudden loss of friends or avoiding social groups
- changes in eating habits

A straight, clean and healthy smile can not only give your child the confidence she needs to embrace her true worth, but can also pave the way toward easier socialization at school, church, or during extracurricular activities. Do your child a favor and talk about her smile and how it might be affecting her.

Beyond that, there's a life ahead of your child. Going to junior high with crooked teeth and a humiliating smile is one thing. Hey, plenty of kids are going to school *without shoes* for heaven's sake. But going to college admission interviews, packing up and heading off to college, going to job interviews, trying to fit into new and anxiety-rich environments at a faraway college or new workplace with a bad smile—and maybe unavoidable bad breath with it—and daytime headaches from nighttime teeth-grinding is a lot more serious.

This isn't *just* a cosmetic issue. Misaligned, crooked teeth equal *significant* medical problems.

Poorly aligned teeth can produce chronic headaches and migraines, contribute to digestive problems because of the inability to properly chew foods, and make getting a decent night's sleep impossible. Perhaps the most dangerous of all: it can foster gum disease. Gum disease has absolute links to diabetes, heart disease, strokes and dementia, as well as, of course, the loss of natural teeth altogether. Orthodontic corrections later in adult life are more difficult; they can be painful, require time off work, and at best, they'll just be embarrassing. *Invisible braces aren't really totally invisible, and you're thirty-eight? Forty-four? Fifty-one? C'mon.*

Uncorrected mouth problems and misaligned teeth make for strangely stretched gums inevitably destined to separate from teeth. This could allow "pockets" for infections and periodontal disease to arise and turn into *very* difficult, painful, and costly problems late in life.

In the teenage years, failure to spend even $4,000 can easily create a $40,000 full mouth restoration case at age forty or fifty, or embarrassing, health-compromising removal of all teeth and use of dentures at age sixty.

Gum disease is serious business. It worsens the risks of and heightens dangers from diabetes, heart disease, strokes, and dementia. Ignoring preteen or teen teeth misalignment may virtually guarantee adult medical problems. If there is a genetic history of any of these medical problems I just named, you only worsen the odds of your son or daughter suffering from them by ignoring or postponing needed orthodontic treatment.

Aside from impacting health, a poorly aligned smile can significantly impact your child's comfort. Headaches, toothaches, sinus problems, dry mouth, snoring, drooling, bad breath, and insomnia are all symptoms of a smile that isn't straight, jaws that aren't aligned, or teeth that are too close together or not quite close enough. Oftentimes, however, the mouth is the last place we check for signs of discomfort, loss of sleep, or even a simple headache.

If your child's pediatrician can't figure out why she's not sleeping well or experiencing headaches or even insomnia for which there seems to be no cause, a simple thirty-minute exam at your local orthodontist could provide a clear solution in no time!

Here is what I'm told by an awful lot of parents:

> "I had wonderful parents, *but* I sure wish they had found a way to afford the braces I needed and gotten me the care I needed when I was a kid, so I didn't grow up to have this bad smile my whole life."

And what I hear from almost every adult patient getting orthodontic treatment and braces is:

> "I had wonderful parents, *but* I sure wish they had found a way to afford the braces I needed and gotten me the care

> I needed when I was a kid, so I didn't grow up to have this bad smile my whole life *and have all these problems now*."

Is this how you want your daughter or son talking about you ten, twenty, or thirty years from now? Is this how you want them remembering their childhood? Your parenting?

If that sounds pretty damned pushy, I admit: it is. I kept it in the book for the very simple reason that this is *truly* what I have heard so much over the years, and I am sincere about letting you reflect on it. All parents want to do the right thing. They don't want to let their children down in any way, and I'm sure you don't either.

You know, parents just about kill themselves over their kids' college, trying their best to guide the decision, trekking around the country on campus visits, worrying over campus culture, or taking on *serious* debt. Every parent understands what many kids can't—that it's not about the few years of college but rather the forty or fifty years afterward.

I assure you, this is the same. It's not about the bad, humiliating smile and bad bite transformed now, for high school. It's about the many, many years to come. They really can't appreciate that now, but *you* can.

No parent wants their child to suffer, either from teeth that actually hurt, headaches you can't explain, insomnia that affects their daily life, or insecurity your child may be feeling because of a crooked or oversized smile. The fact is, your child's formative years are actually the most sensitive for his or her teeth. Now is the time to pay close attention to your child's smile, behavior, peer relationships, and confidence level.

If any or all are lacking, a qualified orthodontist may help give you and your child the peace of mind you both crave.

The Top Five Reasons People Avoid Seeing the Orthodontist

1. **Patients are afraid it's going to hurt.** Pain is the number-one reason most people avoid going to the orthodontist. However, modern technology—and choosing the right orthodontist—can ensure that your child enjoys a comfortable orthodontic experience.
2. **Patients are afraid it's going to cost too much.** Not only are most orthodontic procedures more affordable than ever, but insurance, payment plans, and a variety of other financing options make this all but a moot point for most of my patients. Remember, orthodontists aren't in this to get rich, they're here to make sure your child's teeth, smile, and jaw are aligned to make his or her life better—period! We're not going to let something like price get in the way of creating a better, safer, healthier smile for your child.
3. **Patients are afraid it's going to take too long / they're going to miss too much school or work.** Regardless of the type of orthodontic procedure your child needs, time is of the essence. Modern technology and ease of access allows us to work around your child's school schedule with minimal absences. After initial visits, and barring the actual procedure

itself, most visits and/or adjustments are routine and can take anywhere from ten to twenty minutes.

4. **Patients do not see the need to take action.** Eroding, crooked, or unaligned smiles can take time to happen, but the time to act is now. Orthodontic irregularities don't just heal on their own or disappear if you ignore them. Your child's smile and overall dental health are too important to ignore out of questions of pain, convenience, or even price.

5. **Patients have been treated in the past with an attitude of indifference.** Let's face it, not all doctors are created equal. Every profession has its "bad apples," and to say dentistry is the exception would be to write fiction instead of fact. There is no room for indifference when it comes to your child's healthcare. Find an orthodontic specialist that offers not only state of the art technology for your child, but state of the art service as well. Orthodontic specialists know what it's like to sit in the chair, and should provide every opportunity for patients, especially our younger patients, to feel comfortable, safe, and secure in our care.

Call us at **813-661-1073** or go to **TurkeOrthodontics.com** to schedule your own Customized Smile Analysis.

Chapter Two

Why Do Kids Need Braces?

ARE BRACES SOMETHING CREATED by orthodontists to make money, like Disney and their extra-charge FastPass? Was it a conspiracy from the very start?

Then and now, there may be some overprescribing and premature prescribing by some doctors. There are bad apples in every orchard. And you know the adage: if all he's got is a hammer, everything (and everybody) looks like a nail.

But there is a very legitimate, clinically documented, and 90 percent of the time, clearly visible reason why some kids, as young as eight, *need* orthodontic treatment and care: malocclusion.

Malocclusion is mostly genetic, so if your daughter or son has it, blame their grandparents. It's a fancy-pants term for all things related to misaligned teeth—teeth growing angled, crooked, and into a too-crowded space. It can be a single tooth, a few teeth, or the whole mouth. As I said, it is mostly hereditary, and your kids didn't get to pick their parents out of a Barbie catalog. There can be other causes too, like early, premature loss of primary teeth, chronic thumb-sucking, or even an accident that seemed to leave no lasting effect at its moment in time.

If your child is suffering from any, several, or all of the following early indicators of malocclusion, consider having them addressed by an orthodontic specialist sooner rather than later:

- **Crossbites**: A crossbite occurs when the jaw deviates to one side with an improper fit of the upper and lower teeth from left to right or front to back. Crossbites can lead to worn and chipped teeth, jaw pain, and asymmetric growth of the jaws. Left untreated, the crossbite will require more extensive treatment later in life and significant jaw surgery in the most-severe cases.
- **Thumb-sucking**: Thumb-sucking habits beginning at the age of seven or older should be corrected immediately in order to prevent severe jaw and tooth alignment problems.
- **Speech Problems**: If the teeth are not properly aligned, then it becomes a challenge to properly articulate words.
- **Miscellaneous concerns**: There are several associated issues you should also be looking for as soon as your child turns seven in order to intervene early, including the following:
    - permanent teeth that are growing into the wrong spots
    - severely protruded front teeth at risk for injury or causing teasing at school
    - severe crowding with permanent teeth erupting into poor-quality gum tissue

With any of these situations, we can discuss the pros and cons of early intervention and treatment versus waiting until all the permanent teeth are in for braces. If you are anxious about the appearance of your child's teeth or your child is self-conscious about his or her appearance, early treatment might be the best choice. Not only are most orthodontic problems more difficult to correct later, but self-image and personality inhibition can be hard for a person to leave behind. However, if your child is extremely resistant to braces or is not mature enough to be trusted to care for them, delay may be the better choice. In that case, regularly scheduled orthodontic checkups will be necessary.

Having malocclusion does *not* guarantee a child will need braces. Frankly, this is what worries me about nonspecialists like family dentists substituting themselves for orthodontists, and parents letting it happen. They may easily miss an early diagnosis of malocclusion, when it could have been treated without braces. Or they may leap to braces as the only way to treat all malocclusion. Either way, you and your child lose.

The first question, then, is: does your daughter or son have or show all the signs they are going to have malocclusion? Second, if so, what—of numerous options—should be done about it? Third, when?

To have all these questions answered early, the first full orthodontic exam should occur early in a child's life. I recommend seven or eight, no later than nine, especially if there is family history of malocclusion. With early and periodic exams by an orthodontic specialist, you may avoid your child's need for braces and/or you may prevent years of suffering and embarrassment related to their teeth and smile.

Waiting will have very serious consequences, often requiring more treatment and higher costs later in life. What most parents fail to realize is that these treatment problems are urgent and should be treated as such. If that ship has sailed, the next best time for a full orthodontic exam is tomorrow at three o'clock.

If your son or daughter does need braces—now or at some predictable future time—the outcome of the exam can lead to *sensible* decisions. If not now, treatment to prevent the need can begin, and also, you can begin saving money for braces or other procedures if necessary later on in your child's life. There is no tooth fairy coming to leave a few thousand dollars underneath his pillow or yours. But if the need must be met three years from now, skipping one Starbucks run a week for those three years can make a hefty dent in the bill to come. Utilizing a Health Savings Account or Flex Spending Account can help, as well. How to fund orthodontic treatment is discussed later in the book.

Let me be emphatically clear. I am *not* in the business of putting braces on any child who doesn't need braces. My office is *not* a braces store. I'm in the business of helping kids and families get the right orthodontic treatment if any is needed, get the right braces if any are needed, and have as perfect a smile and as few oral health problems as possible. I make sure my patients are informed—that's why I wrote this book. In my office, you're never told what to do. You're provided with real information, no medical jargon, plain English, "reasons why," and options. You probably know the term "God complex," referring to a person who acts like he's God—imperious, brusque, and deliberately intimidating to squash questions. You will *not* get that kind of treatment here, from me or anyone on my team.

Kids do need braces, but not all kids and certainly not the same braces for all. Some kids are better served by other orthodontic treatments instead of or before braces. We will collaborate, you and I, to figure out what is or isn't needed and what options are best if there is a need for your child.

Call us at **813-661-1073** or go to **TurkeOrthodontics.com** to schedule your own Customized Smile Analysis.

Chapter Three

Why Not Just a Dentist? Why an Orthodontist?

YOU UNDOUBTEDLY ALREADY have a dentist.

Gee, isn't seeing an orthodontist going to cost a lot more?

I'm busy. More appointments?

Do I really need to get orthodontic checkups for my kids?

Don't worry, these are all reasonable questions! It is true that, today, quite a few dentists dance over into our territory, and although they're *not* permitted to claim they're the same as orthodontists or provide orthodontic treatment (beware of any who do), they're able to do things like provide Invisalign and other braces. This can be confusing. Here are the facts.

All orthodontists are dentists and we all graduate from the same dental schools. True enough. But that's where it stops for dentists. Orthodontists go to school for an additional two to three years to become credentialed specialists at diagnosing and providing the best treatment for conditions like:

- difficulties chewing or biting
- constant biting into the cheek, gums, or roof of the mouth
- teeth that meet abnormally or don't meet at all
- teeth grinding or clenching
- crowded, misplaced, or blocked out teeth
- early or late loss of teeth
- teeth grown in badly
- teeth that protrude
- embarrassing personal appearance due to teeth
- facial imbalances
- teeth or jaw misalignment, TMJ
- chronic headaches and migraine
- poor sleep
- speech difficulties (that may never be outgrown or may develop later)

These are *not* dental care issues. They are orthodontic issues.

For *some* things, a generalist or jack-of-all-trades will do. For other things, you know it's smart to seek out the best specialist you can afford. For example, if all your income is in a single W-2 from one employer and you have simple, ordinary deductions, getting your taxes prepared for the cheapest fee at the seasonal H&R Block office that opens up in your neighborhood shopping center is probably fine. But if you have W-2, 1099, and investment income from real estate, depreciation on real estate in several states, own stocks, and you raise iguanas as a money hobby, you're going to get yourself a really good accountant, probably a CPA. If you need the simplest will, leaving everything first to spouse or second to daughter may be okay. But if you are of some means and have several children and maybe also grandchildren as well as charities, you're going to need to see an *estate planning* attorney, not just any attorney—though they all went to the same law schools—but *a specialist in estate planning.*

This is no different.

There are a few things to keep in mind when differentiating between a general dentist and an orthodontic specialist.

First, generalists, or jacks-of-all-trades, tend to work with one-size-fits-all, off-the-rack, standardized solutions. They may be limited to doing only what the computer dictates that they do, without bringing expertise and expert judgment to bear. They're often working with products from only one provider, without being able to select from a full range of options that would work best for you. Specialists, instead, tend to individually and carefully diagnose needs and provide personalized solutions.

Second, generalists and their use of inexpertly applied, standardized solutions tend to be cheaper than the fees of a specialist, but that also places economic pressure on them to do the treatment as quickly and simply as possible, because they've "cut it thin."

In this case, it's worth remembering that the treatment provided has permanent, lifelong, and life-impacting consequences. This concerns your health, future dental or jaw alignment or misalignment issues affecting quality of sleep (which can affect weight, even onset and management of type 2 diabetes and heart disease), as well as self-esteem and social and career success.

> **General Dentist.** A general dentist gives routine checkups, preventative measures, cleans teeth, and fixes cavities. They may not start seeing children until they are seven to ten years old.
>
> **Pediatric Dentist.** A pediatric dentist has two to three years of specialized education beyond dental school. They specialize in providing dental care to children and adolescents, offering checkups, preventative measures, cleanings, and cavities.
>
> **Orthodontist.** An orthodontist has two to three years of specialized education beyond dental school and is an expert at straightening teeth and aligning the jaws. They assess patients and determine the best treatment routes and procedures that need to be taken.

If you can, you want to choose an orthodontist for orthodontic care.

You may ask, *how do I know my doctor is an orthodontist?* It's a good question and a critical one to ask as you seek additional treatment for your child's dental issues.

Only orthodontists can belong to the American Association of Orthodontists (AAO). If you're looking for a local orthodontist, go online and visit **www.braces.org** to find a specialist in your area. This website features not only a searchable database of orthodontists but educational tips, answers and resources to help you on your quest for your child's healthiest smile!

Alternatively, you can ask your doctor if he or she has completed a two- to three-year residency in orthodontics and check with your state dental board to follow up on his reply. Dentists and orthodontists in most states will be registered differently with the dental board.

Do your homework; be a "dental detective" while on the hunt for such vital information. Look for the words "dental specialist in orthodontics," or ask your general dentist for a referral to a specialist. In urban and suburban areas, it will take minimal effort to find a specialist. In more remote, rural locations, your search might take you to another city or town. Don't be afraid to ask your dentist if an orthodontist travels to your town every month to see patients. There's a chance an orthodontist from a larger city comes to your town and works out of another dental office once or twice per month. Looking around can save valuable driving time and money.

One note: there is no disrespect between orthodontists and dentists. As a matter of fact, many orthodontic patients are referred by their dentists. These are great, capable, and caring professionals who know where their expertise begins and ends, and who do not let ego or income opportunity step in front of what they know is best for their patients. Just as the family doctor refers his patients with possible or significant heart disease issues to a cardiologist, and if need be, the cardiologist refers to a surgeon, the best dentists refer patients with orthodontic needs to orthodontists. Orthodontists are required to take two to three years of university education beyond dental school and additional continuing clinical education every year. They must also invest in state-of-the-art technology for their offices (not found in dental offices)—*all for a good reason.*

Even though we orthodontists have the education and training to perform general dentist procedures, we don't. We specialize.

Call us at **813-661-1073** or go to **TurkeOrthodontics.com** to schedule your own Customized Smile Analysis.

Chapter Four

How to Choose Your Orthodontist

This is something you want to be sure about.

Here are a few suggestions to consider when selecting an orthodontist that will be the best fit for you.

1. Are they a specialist?

Orthodontists are specially trained dentists who take on several extra years of training in order to "straighten teeth," usually by affixing braces to the patient's teeth. You might say we specialize in smiles. Orthodontists also perform dentofacial orthopedics. This is a fancy way to describe how we normalize the structure of a patient's jawbones in order to repair any imbalance in their face. All orthodontists are dentists, but only 6 percent of dentists are orthodontists. Look for the seal of the American Association of Orthodontists (AAO). Only orthodontic specialists can belong to the AAO.

2. Do they have a great reputation?

How many years have the Orthodontist's been in practice, and what are their patients saying about the experience. How involved are they in investing and advancing the future of their profession. A few ways to evaluate their involvement is if they are faculty at a dental school or residency program, a published author, or a speaker in their field.

3. Do they treat adults?

Orthodontics is not just for kids! It's important that your orthodontist can treat patients of all ages. Many adults are finding out how a healthy and attractive smile is important to their health and the way they feel about themselves. Others choose to avoid a lifetime of crooked teeth for health concerns or problems with their bite.

4. Do they provide the first visit free of charge?

Most orthodontists offer free examinations for new patients so you and your family can get expert advice about treatment needs, options, and timing before making this important investment. During your first exam and consultation be sure your questions are answered, your concerns are addressed, and you are educated about all of your treatment options. The orthodontist should include digital x-rays during the exam at no charge.

5. Are they using the latest technology and treatment options available?

Orthodontics today differs a great deal from years past. Technology has dramatically increased the precision with which we move teeth and shorten treatment time. Today's advanced braces systems have made treatment far more efficient and comfortable. Clear braces offer a cosmetically pleasing alternative, while Invisalign offers patients an entirely brace-free option. Did you know that Invisalign also has a special treatment system just for teens?

Ultimately, you get the best treatment available when you choose us.

6. Does their quoted fee include retainers?

Each orthodontic office has its own fee schedules, and doctors often charge differently for procedures. All orthodontists should offer you a contract that clearly spells out the expenses for your child's treatment before it begins.

Throughout the orthodontic industry, it's common to find out about retainer fees after you start treatment. You should ask your orthodontist about what retainers cost and also if there are any other hidden fees.

7. Are they flexible with payment options?

Once you are comfortable and you know specifically which orthodontist you want to treat you or your child, the next question is typically, "How much is this going to cost and how am I going to pay for this?"

We help you understand different payment options from maximizing the most insurance benefits to flex spending accounts to even interest-free payment plans. During the initial exam and complimentary consultation, we will answer all of your questions, including those about our typical cost of braces and the variety of payment options available.

How to Know What Questions to Ask

I've really thought through the questions most parents and patients have—not just the ones they ask, but the ones they don't. This book attempts to cover them all, but again, this is a *personal* matter. The best questions to ask are the ones that matter most to you and your child.

I hope not, but you may be in a position that absolutely requires you to get the minimum essential treatment for the lowest cost. If so, your most important questions are going to be about those kinds of options and about price, and nothing else.

If, however, you are able to make your decision about who you should trust with your child's oral health and smile by many factors, we've included a "What Is Most Important to You?" quiz from Excellence In Orthodontics on the following pages. As you'll see, there are fourteen different items to consider and rank in importance to you. Any can become the questions you ask me and my team or any other orthodontist.

Incidentally, Excellence In Orthodontics is a national organization for exceptionally successful orthodontists leading the field in both clinical and patient care and patient/parent (client) service excellence. We all subscribe to a pledge of very high standards and hold each other accountable. You can learn more at ExcellenceInOrthdontics.org.

If you have a specific question not answered anywhere in this book, or have a personal and confidential question, you can—with complete assurance of privacy and courtesy—email helloturkebn@verizon.net or call Dr. Eric Turke at 813-661-1073.

There is also a FAQ section at the back of this book.

Of course, a perfect opportunity to get questions answered—yours and your son's or daughter's—is at your exam appointment.

Call us at **813-661-1073** or go to **TurkeOrthodontics.com** to schedule your own Customized Smile Analysis.

What Is Most Important to You?

Directions: For each **Key Item** below, rank its importance to you from 1 to 5. Then check off whether each type of provider provides that item. When you're done with all 14 Key Items, add up your rankings and review what your final score means about choosing an orthodontist.

	Key Items to Consider in Selecting Your Orthodontist	**Rank How Important Each Item Is to You** in Selecting Your Orthodontist 1 – Not Important, 5 – Very Important	**Check Off If Provided** Turke Orthodontics	Other Provider	Other Provider
1	Orthodontist and staff committed to expert, thorough diagnosis, and prescription of the best treatment plan customized for my son or daughter	1 2 3 4 5	✓		
2	Avoiding extractions (if possible)	1 2 3 4 5	✓		
3	Avoiding having to wear headgear with braces (if possible)	1 2 3 4 5	✓		
4	Avoiding "metal-mouth" braces (if possible) or utilizing the new type of "invisible" braces	1 2 3 4 5	✓		
5	Having a healthy, pleasing smile that will last a lifetime and protect optimum dental health (not just having straightened teeth)	1 2 3 4 5	✓		
6	Pain-free treatment	1 2 3 4 5	✓		
7	Orthodontist utilizes the most modern, advanced, and proven technology, including computer-aided design and fitting	1 2 3 4 5	✓		
8	Orthodontists and team actively involved in continuing clinical education	1 2 3 4 5	✓		
9	Reducing treatment time to a minimum without compromising results (including total length of treatment term and number of office visits)	1 2 3 4 5	✓		
10	Availability of after-school or after-work appointment options	1 2 3 4 5	✓		
11	Treatment coordinator is knowledgeable about insurance coverage and is able to offer flexible payment plans	1 2 3 4 5	✓		

12	Getting the best overall value factoring in thorough diagnosis, customized care, and concern with lifetime health and well-being—not just the cheapest fee	1 2 3 4 5	✓		
13	Lifetime guarantee	1 2 3 4 5	✓		
14	Orthodontist and team committed to excellence in orthodontics and customer service for both patients and parents	1 2 3 4 5	✓		
Total of Your Rankings					

What Your Score Means

50-70 There is no doubt. Turke Orthodontics is the right choice for you and your family! It is clear that you place a high value on a comprehensive, "best" approach.

43-49 You are probably also going to be happiest with Turke Orthodontics, rather than any other alternative. But this score suggests you aren't completely sure and have some unanswered questions or concerns. Your doctor and the practice's treatment coordinator want no lingering uncertainties on your part, and want to address any and every question. Don't keep anything to yourself. Please ask.

42 or less Frankly, you may not value the advanced, sophisticated level of clinical care and customer service provided at Turke Orthodontics. Cost may be much more important to you than other factors, or very basic service may be all you feel you need. It's perfectly okay. If you choose to shop around, be sure to use this checklist in evaluating other options. Remember, you do want everything right the first time, and you want error-free orthodontics at a minimum.

Chapter Five

How to Get More Information

THERE ARE SEVERAL WAYS to get information about our orthodontic practice. First, visit our website (Turke-Orthodontics.com). It is interesting, easy to use, and very informative about our practice. Secondly, I want to address the ways I don't recommend.

I don't recommend Yelp. Yelp is, unfortunately, not at all what it seems, and is frequently the subject of lawsuits from business owners, under regulatory scrutiny centered around the poorly policed manipulation of reviews, and has even been accused of the flooding of fake reviews—by "bots" no less! Some companies can use Yelp as competitive warfare while other companies turn around and sell the business owner under negative-review-assault "reputation management services." So, beware! Get the information you need from truly trusted sources.

Google can also be deceptive, though I admit it can be a valuable starting point. Rankings are manipulated by advertisements, websites, YouTube content, and what's called SEO, or search engine optimization. The only thing you know for sure about dentists or orthodontists who come up at the top in Google rankings in your community is that they are good at SEO or, more likely, good at paying somebody who is good at SEO. They're willing to spend money and willing to create a lot of content. Does that equate to certainty of the best diagnostic expertise, treatment, patient care, and customer service? Sometimes. Sometimes not.

So, first, the best thing to do is make certain you get all your questions answered by the orthodontist. My own goal in this is to have every patient and every patient's parent feel comfortable with the treatment plan in order to minimize anxiety.

Second, visit ExcellenceInOrthodontics.org. This is an organization of carefully chosen orthodontists joined together to provide carefully curated, vetted, authoritative, accurate, and understandable patient and parent information, hence its name. This can definitely help you decide on the questions you want answers to.

Finally, if you have a quick follow-up visit scheduled, these are wonderful opportunities to either ask questions you may have missed the first time, or to get further details from your orthodontist directly.

Now that we know where to get your most burning orthodontic questions answered, here are some simple tips I've amassed over the years to help you easily and effectively get the information you need:

How to Get Your Questions Answered

Make a list. The easiest way to get what you want is to know it in advance. Make a list of the various questions you have when they arise so you can quickly and easily go down the list to assure you've got the right answers for the right questions.

Bring it with you. Take the list with you when you go for your child's orthodontist visit. This way you have the questions at hand at the right place at the right time. If you're calling in to get answers, you can also have the list ready and tick off one question for every answer you receive.

Record the answers. If your orthodontist, or their receptionist, speaks too fast or you can't keep up while writing the answers down, why not record them? Your cell phone likely has a "record" feature, and if not, there are many affordable micro-recorders on the market today.

Double-check. Finally, make sure you have the right answer by double-checking with your orthodontist or their receptionist or assistant.

Knowing where to find the information you need is only half the battle; follow these tips and you'll know how to get what you're looking for as well.

Read this book. This book is very informative and has what every parent needs to know about orthodontics. This book will also give you insights into how Dr. Turke fixes smiles and how these changed smiles can indeed change lives!

Regardless of how many questions you have, or your comfort level with technology, phone calls, or in-person visits, your orthodontist should offer an option that fits your schedule and makes all your unresolved issues crystal clear.

Call us at **813-661-1073** or go to **TurkeOrthodontics.com** to schedule your own Customized Smile Analysis.

Chapter Six

How to Pay For Orthodontic Treatment and Braces

YOU MAY HAVE NEVER needed braces. Or you may have needed them and gotten them. Or you may be among the tens of thousands of people in our generation who needed them but did not get them, perhaps because your family decided they couldn't afford them. Maybe they didn't consider it a priority and probably underestimated the lifelong results of the decision. You may not only have lived with a "hide your smile" habit unnecessarily, but you may have developed chronic jaw pain and headaches, difficulty chewing, or even periodontal disease that could have been prevented.

Regardless of which group you're in—and I hope it's not the third—I hope you will be making the best choices for your son or daughter today, without being hamstrung just by the finances. Truth is, parents pay out the same cost for a number of different things not nearly as vital as health or emotional well-being without blinking, mostly because it's paid in installments or just never really *considered*, like the monthly cost for minutes/data on mobile devices, added up for a year or two. The additional insurance cost and other costs when the teenager gets his driver's permit; after all, what's the choice? The cost of braces leaps up and stands there, all at one time. So, it can seem big. And it tempts thoughts of, "maybe later," or, "is this really necessary?"

I hope in the prior chapters I have succeeded at getting the "is it really necessary?" question erased. If there is visible need or if expert examination by an orthodontist and his explanation of what he finds can show you say it is advisable, it *is* necessary! It won't fix itself. It will probably get worse. It plagues a person's health, emotional well-being, social life, and career. It can link to very serious medical problems. *Necessary* is not really debatable.

Now let's tackle the ugly matter of the money.

I say "ugly" because nobody really likes talking about this. Most orthodontists are nervous about it. Parents are uncomfortable with it. If there is a financial obstacle to treatment, most people are reluctant to admit it, offer other excuses, and then can't be helped by the doctor. I think we have to trust each other. With me, this discussion is entirely confidential, in a "safe zone." Orthodontists are not Martians, by the way; *we* have kids, college tuitions that loom, and family budgets.

What Is a Reasonable Fee and Cost?

A complete, comprehensive treatment program, including braces, can cost anywhere from $4,000 to $10,000 or so. Most fall in between. Adjusted for inflation, these prices are actually *less than* braces decades ago, while the technology and quality has advanced. In costs it can prevent later, it's a bona fide bargain. TMJ treatments are expensive.

Cosmetic dentistry work is expensive. Migraine headache drugs are expensive and have side effects.

For this investment, you will be getting the carefully selected, personalized solution to your child's irregularities and problems, prescribed using state-of-the-art digital technology along with the expertise of a specialist, and considerate, compassionate care from start to finish. Your investment in orthodontic treatment can help change you or your child's life by gaining confidence in their smile and improving their health and self esteem.

In this case, the $4,000 to $10,000 range is seen as perfectly reasonable by the overwhelming majority of parents that I talk to. Each year, we provide braces of one kind or another to countless patients. Even parents who shook their heads at the cost to start with tell me afterward that having witnessed everything we do to get the absolute best obtainable results, and seeing the outcome itself, they feel undercharged.

While it's never easy to part with such a sum, people do it every day for all sorts of less important things, like their new designer handbag, golf vacation, or suite of living room furniture. They'll pay for it outright or with their favorite credit card (getting the reward points in the bargain). If you put the orthodontic treatment program including braces on a typical credit card at the interest in play as I write this, and you choose to make only the minimum required monthly payment, your monthly payments will be relatively small. Even tight budgets can accommodate this *when it is really important.* It's less than most families pay for their cable and streaming entertainment. For many, if they got all their Starbucks stops consolidated into one monthly bill, it would be more than this!

Health Spending Accounts (HSA) / Flex Spending Accounts (FSA)

The HSA allows you to set aside *pre-tax* dollars to be used for certain medical and health expenses for you or your family. They exist although restricted under the Affordable Care Act (Obamacare) as it stood in July of 2017. By the time you read this, the opportunity may have been expanded, as President Trump suggested. In any case, if you have accumulated money in an HSA, you can probably spend it on orthodontic treatment. If you don't have an HSA, you might want to start one. Information can be found online about existing or new accounts and their rules of use, at www.healthcare.gov.

Other kinds of FSAs are typically set up through your place of employment and similarly enable you to set aside pre-tax dollars for medical expenses. Sometimes, employers match contributions. Again, you can almost certainly tap funds from your FSA for your child's orthodontic care. Check with your employer about this.

If you have a tax accountant, you may want to consult with him about your HSA or FSA.

> **TIP**: How can you make the most out of your employer's flex-pay plan? First, make sure you understand how it works. Second, set aside flex-spending dollars in advance of need, and if possible, make the maximum contributions. Many employers allow higher limits than you'd think without asking, as much as $2,500 to $5,000 per year. Be aware of "family status changes" allowed by your plan that may enable you to change the amount being moved pre-tax from

your paychecks to your account anytime during the year rather than just once at the first of the year—so you could bump up the amount in months before the first orthodontic treatment. IMPORTANT: be aware of the balance and the loss of unused funds. In most cases, if you do not use these funds, you lose them, year to year. You usually have three months after the end of the calendar year to submit claims for eligible expenses from the previous year.

Insurance

These days, there are as many different types of insurance plans as there are patients in my office. I can't possibly speak to your unique and personal insurance policy without seeing it first but, in general, my experience tells me that "most" insurance policies cover "some" of your orthodontic expenses.

I realize that answer sounds very vague, but here are a couple of variables you need to answer before an insurance agent can help you determine what, how long, and how many procedures fall under your insurance:

- the type of procedure (braces, Invisalign, etc.)
- the duration of the procedure (two months, six months, a year, etc.)
- the cause of the procedure (a patient presenting with pain, a parent's concern, traumatic injury or accident, congenital birth defect like cleft lip or palate, etc.)

- the nature of the procedure (to correct pain/discomfort, cosmetic, etc.)

I can only partially answer this question, but talking to your insurance agent will help you get the right answers you need.

> **TIP**: Keep an insurance journal of every interaction with your carrier. Write down the date, time of call, name of the person you contacted, and the exact instructions or recommendations following the call. Later, if your insurance company doesn't remember what they told you, you'll have it accurately written down. If they still don't remember, ask them to pull the recorded audio tape from your previous call, so that you can accurately "remind" them of exactly what they told you.

Loans

If you qualify, we offer Care Credit, which can provide an unsecured, signature-only loan for the treatment program, with repayment over twelve to sixty months. You don't need to go anywhere else to apply or do paperwork; we can take care of it in my office.

If you have equity in your home, the lowest-cost loan option may be a home equity line of credit or second mortgage. See your own bank, or check out RocketMortgage at rocket.quickenloans.com. As of this writing, mortgage interest is at record lows.

Obviously, a private loan from a family member can be the easiest option. A lot of preteens' and teens' important orthodontic care is financed at the Bank of Grandma and Grandpa.

If the other options are difficult or unavailable, we will set up a reasonable payment plan with a comfortable monthly payment.

What If You Really, Really Can't Afford Braces?

I have compiled a list of eighteen ways you may be able to substantially reduce the cost of braces. Frankly, some of them are less than ideal, and most are not available through my office, but they could be helpful if your back is really up against a financial wall.

1. **See if your local dental school has an orthodontic program.** The treatment at such institutions is supervised by board-certified orthodontists (most of whom practice in the surrounding area). While you might spend a little more time in the chair as a teaching case, if you have the time, it might be well worth the wait because you can sometimes save up to *half the cost of traditional braces.*
2. **Ask your insurance plans when they send out their fee schedules to participating providers.** If the insurance company updates their fees or the orthodontist raises his or her fees to keep up with the cost of inflation, it might be around November in preparation for the next year.
3. **See your dentist every four to six months.** While you're wearing your braces, the extra cleaning each year can prevent tooth decay, a costly item to repair.
4. **Get your flex spending dollars in order with your employer.** If you set money aside in a flex plan, it may be

"tax-free," but it comes with some stipulations: namely, you have to use it before the end of the year or else you lose it.

5. **See if you can get a second set of retainers from your orthodontist at the end of treatment.** Sometimes getting two sets of retainers at the same time can be cheaper than buying a second set later in life when you lose or break your first set.

6. **See if your husband or wife has an insurance plan that covers braces.** Be sure to enroll in the plan with enough time to spare before your child needs braces, so that the procedure is not denied by your insurance company due to a waiting period.

7. **Got taxes?** Good! Why not use your tax refund to help pay for treatment in full and ask for a courtesy on the average fees associated with financing a full orthodontic case? In some areas, you can save as much as 10 percent on the cost of braces by simply saving your pennies and paying the entire bill at once, up front.

8. **Ask for more flexible financing through a third-party credit company, through CareCredit, or by using in-house financing through your orthodontist.** Most orthodontists will accept a reasonable down payment and split the remaining amount into easy monthly payments for your convenience. With automated withdrawals from a credit card, you might be able to stretch the monthly payments out over a longer period to make each payment lower. Just don't be shocked if your orthodontist asks you to approve a credit check. A little homework up front can

be well worth the effort when your monthly orthodontic bill is lower than your cell phone bill!

Call us at **813-661-1073** or go to **TurkeOrthodontics.com** to schedule your own Customized Smile Analysis.

Chapter Seven

What Are the Treatment Options?

IF YOUR CHILD IS ready for orthodontic care, one of the first discussions to have with your orthodontist is which procedure is right for him or her; there might be more options than you had ever imagined.

If you're like most people, you associate orthodontists with braces, but these days, that is just one arm of what I or any orthodontist does. Here are some of the services most orthodontists will provide their patients with during the course of routine treatment:

- early treatment and growth modification
- customized appliances designed uniquely for each patient
- metal, tie-free braces
- Invisalign clear removable aligners
- clear braces

- expanders to match jaw size and tooth size
- habit appliances to eliminate thumb sucking
- space maintainers
- retainers to prevent crowding and shifting of teeth
- headgear to help correct jaw alignment
- functional appliances to help improve facial balance

While many of these services may seem self-explanatory to you, several will probably not. In the following pages, I will try to elaborate on several of them, including:

- crossbite correction
- metal braces
- clear braces
- Invisalign

Crossbite Correction

As your child's teeth begin to grow in, there's a *lot* more at work than mere gum lines, tooth fairies, and molar size. How the jaw is shaped, when it develops, and even how "normally" it develops can all affect the placement and comfort of your child's teeth.

When the upper and lower teeth grow at different rates, or even when the lower jaw grows disproportionately with the upper jaw, something known as a "crossbite" can occur.

Your child might have a crossbite if, for instance, the lower jaw is out of line with the upper jaw (kind of like a box that won't close right because one of the hinges is bent).

Or perhaps on the right side of your child's mouth, the lower teeth "stick out" a little farther than the top teeth, making the upper teeth on that side overlap in turn.

Or maybe your child's upper and lower jaws are out of alignment so instead of the top and bottom front teeth meeting "naturally" as they should, the front teeth fall somewhat behind the lower teeth. This would be the reverse of an overbite.

As you might imagine, any or all of these developments can lead to short- and long-term discomfort and functional bite problems for your child.

How, When, and Why Crossbites Form

You might be amazed to find out how many ways a crossbite can form as your child grows and develops during his or her formative years. Heredity is one key to jaw growth, or alignment, as is the size of your child's developing jaw.

Another factor that can contribute to the development of a potential crossbite is if it takes your child too long to lose his or her baby teeth. In some extreme cases, in fact, if it takes too long for your child to lose his baby teeth, another set of teeth can grow in behind them, throwing the alignment off and contributing to a crossbite.

Believe it or not, something as basic as whether your child breathes through her nose or her mouth can also contribute to a crossbite. While most children breathe through their noses, some children develop a habit early on of breathing through their mouths instead.

In children who breathe through their noses while they're sleeping, the tongue naturally rests on the roof of the mouth, promoting natural and proper upper jaw growth. When young children breathe through their mouths, however, the tongue relocates from the roof of the mouth to the bottom, removing that extra support and potentially contributing to reduced upper jaw bone growth; this can create the crossbite we spoke of previously.

How Can I Spot a Crossbite?

Although it sounds severe, and even painful from the description provided earlier, the effects of a crossbite can take time to manifest themselves. Still, here are some of the telltale signs your child might be cultivating, or already suffering from, a crossbite:

- snoring
- difficulty breathing
- chewing on one side of the mouth or the other
- signs of an underbite
- if your child's chin seems "off center" or disproportionate

How, When, and Why to Correct a Crossbite

Where should you start looking for treatment if you're concerned about your child's jaw development after reading this section? If you suspect your child might have a crossbite, call our office for a complimentary evaluation.

There are many possible treatments available for a crossbite, and your orthodontist can work with you closely to make the right and specific decisions for you and your child.

When should you start? I believe you know my standard answer when it comes to questions like this one: *as early as possible*! The same way an auto mechanic would tell you to take care of that oil leak, bulging tire, or faulty timing belt sooner rather than later, myself and my colleagues in orthodontics will always favor early treatment to later.

Crossbites are often closely linked with other orthodontic issues, such as teeth alignment, jaw size, and growth, so naturally, the sooner you address any or all of these issues, the better.

Finally, why should you address a crossbite? Crossbites can lead to pain, discomfort, and a lack of confidence as your child begins to feel insecure or even ostracized because of this very treatable, very normal series of jaw and teeth developments.

Not only can crossbites become physically uncomfortable if left untreated, but if the misalignment or root cause of the bite isn't fixed early in childhood, then the child's appearance and, ultimately, confidence could be affected as the crossbite becomes more pronounced in adolescence.

Metal Braces

The fact is, metal braces still have a valued place in the orthodontic world, and despite advances and breakthroughs of products like Invisalign and even clear braces, they aren't going extinct anytime soon! This is because metal braces are very strong and can withstand most types of treatment. In our office, we use the latest in advanced technology to provide metal braces that are smaller, sleeker, and more polished than ever before.

"Dr. Turke has put braces on 3 of our children and we are back with a fourth. Our experience has been great every time. None of our children have had any problems with their teeth since their braces have come off. Dr. Turke has been quick to see us and fix any issues that we have had. I have recommended many people to Dr. Turke over the years."

—STEVEN & ARLEEN C.

Clear Braces

Adults and teenagers like to choose ceramic because they "blend in" with the teeth and are less noticeable than metal. These are the type of braces actor Tom Cruise had.

Adult Orthodontics

It's not uncommon for individuals who have undergone orthodontic treatment earlier in life to find their teeth have drifted out of alignment over the years. Most adults won't think twice about bleaching their teeth to roll back the effects of time. Yet few think about the role orthodontics can play.

Adults of all ages can enjoy the same cosmetic and health benefits of properly aligned teeth with our modern technology available in our office.

Improperly aligned teeth can do more than undermine your confidence. They can make proper cleaning and brushing more difficult, contribute to enamel loss, and even set the stage for more significant problems down the road. Orthodontic treatment can give you that smile you've been waiting for to live a healthier, happier lifestyle.

The Solution Is Clear

Orthodontists believe every individual has the right to live their life with a smile they truly love, particularly children. Healthy, straight, and attractive smiles make your child happier and more self-confident. And isn't that what we all want for them?

New orthodontic technology helps you achieve the smile of your dreams faster, easier, and more discretely than you ever imagined. Embrace the confidence that comes with beautifully aligned teeth and put your smile on display. Schedule a consultation and ask if orthodontic treatment is right for you.

By utilizing modern technology in our appliances and braces, your treatment can proceed faster with fewer follow-up visits than older, traditional fixed wire braces.

Invisalign

Invisalign is a widely advertised, well-known, and popular orthodontic product, and kids often know about it and ask parents and doctors for it by name. For many, it's as good an option as any other and sometimes even the best option.

Invisalign uses advanced, proprietary 3-D computer-imaging technology to "map" the entire span of treatment, from the present teeth alignment to the desired positioning, alignment, and smile. Clear aligners are custom made and based on the 3-D imaging. Invisalign has many features that have helped make it such a popular choice. The aligners are removable, even before a snack or meal as well as for general hygiene. There are no metal brackets or wires. Office visits for adjustments throughout the treatment program are fast, easy and painless. The thermoplastic aligners are virtually invisible. Over four million patients have been treated with Invisalign, and there is a special Invisalign system for teens.

Because Invisalign is computer mapped, there's sometimes the idea that anybody can install Invisalign and that all practitioners using Invisalign are the same. I have an important warning about this: during each stage of the complete treatment, only certain teeth are allowed to move. Which teeth move in what order, and the amount of time (days/weeks) needed for each successive set of aligners differs for each patient. *This* is what you rely on an expert orthodontist specializing in pediatric and juvenile care to decide. At the start, we determine whether your son or daughter is a good candidate for the Invisalign approach, or if they would be better served with different braces. You have to rely on *somebody* to tell you. I promise you, there are kids who've been hurried to Invisalign who were not good candidates for it.

Invisalign Teen

Much like the standard adult version, the Invisalign Teen System lets you do it the modern, hygienic way. Your new smile is created with the most innovative technology—a series of clear aligners that are custom-fit to your teeth.

The first thing you should know is that an average treatment takes about a year. Plus, your treatment can begin even if you don't have all of your permanent teeth. Invisalign Teen was designed to meet your needs.

Invisalign Teen aligners will snap on your child's teeth easily. They are comfortable and practically invisible. Invisalign Teen allows for permanent teeth to grow gently while continuously moving teeth in small increments. Aligners are worn for about one to two weeks and then swapped for a new pair.

Invisalign Teen aligners have a "Blue Dot Wear Indicator," designed to show an estimation of wear time. The dot is designed to fade until it's clear over a one- to two-week period if you wear your aligners properly (meaning for twenty to twenty-two hours every day).

Invisalign Teen is designed to custom-fit to your child's teeth and go with his or her lifestyle. During your treatment, your child can keep smiling, playing sports, eating what he or she wants, and brushing and flossing normally because the aligners are removable. Plus, unlike traditional braces, the aligners are made of smooth plastic and move teeth gradually.

After your child's Invisalign Teen treatment, you may find his or her self-confidence boosted by their new smile and the change in their appearance. Some people even feel that way during the treatment. As you know, smiling has many benefits. It can help your child make a strong impression in lots of different social situations—at school, at work, or at a party.

Invisalign Teen really works. It helps correct a broad range of dental and orthodontic issues. You can get a confident smile without metal bands, brackets, or wires. It works on many kinds of conditions, including overly crowded or widely spaced teeth, crossbites, overbites, and underbites.

We've used Invisalign to successfully transform the smiles of many patients, but we do not prescribe it to everybody. After all, *popularity* should not govern medical care!

Trustworthy, Objective Advice

Our office is *not* "in the pocket of" or obligated to any of these providers of different braces products and technologies. We select and recommend what we believe is *the* most appropriate and beneficial choice for your child. We are happy to discuss the pros and cons of different ones, if your child has heart set on, say, Invisalign, because that's what a friend has, or based on information you've obtained.

The number-one rule here is: what is absolutely best for the patient?

Call us at **813-661-1073** or go to **TurkeOrthodontics.com** to schedule your own Customized Smile Analysis.

Chapter Eight

How Difficult Is Living with Braces

REMEMBER, THIS ISN'T 1982. Or 1992. Today's braces aren't anything like yours if you had them decades ago. Today's orthodontic care is far more advanced, more sophisticated, and more patient-centered than any prior generation has experienced. If you had traditional metal braces twenty years or so ago, you experienced medieval torture. The dungeon is gone too, replaced by ultra-modern, comfortable, and patient-friendly offices. Out of the dark, into the light!

Living with braces is *not* going to be anywhere near as difficult as you might imagine.

Let's look at a few specific concerns.

Brushing and Hygiene

Modern braces, whether they're metal, flexible, or "invisible," are all actually made to fit the individual and facilitate easy, painless, thorough brushing. This means your child brushes pretty much the same as he would if he didn't have braces.

Here are some simple tips you can share with your child for the best results when brushing with braces on:

- Brush your teeth with a soft nylon toothbrush after each time you eat and before bed.
- Brush, rinse, and look; if you find any areas that are not clean, brush them again.
- Brush your gums as you brush your teeth (massage and stimulate).
- Take extra care in the area between the gums and the braces because food caught and left there can cause swollen gums, cavities, discomfort, and permanent teeth stains.
- If no toothpaste is available, brush without.
- If you are unable to brush, rinse your mouth vigorously with water.
- Replace your old toothbrush when it gets worn out.
- It's absolutely essential you continue regular visits to your family dentist for checkups and cleanings throughout your orthodontic treatment!

Depending on the age of your child, you, the parent, may need to supervise the first few brushings with the braces in place. You should *not* have a whining, resistant, difficult child on your hands because of any of this. It's like learning to ride a bike or sew. The more you do it, the easier it becomes. In the same way, brushing and flossing with your orthodontic appliances just takes a bit of time and practice.

Forbidden Foods Your Child Must Avoid

After your child's orthodontic appliance/braces have been placed, the teeth are usually "tender" and sensitive for as few as three to as many as ten days: a *short* time. During these few days, softer foods are recommended: soups, macaroni, spaghetti, eggs, fish, Jell-O, yogurt. As needed, Tylenol or Advil are adequate in relieving any discomfort, taken an hour or so before eating.[2] Warm saltwater rinses can be helpful. We also provide a "soft white wax" that can be used like a band-aid to be placed over any rough corners of the braces. It can also be used to cover any wires that might become displaced in the event of a sporting accident or injury until the patient can come into our office.

For the entire duration of the braces being in place, I'd advise you to stay away from hard and sticky foods that can damage braces and may lengthen the time they have to be worn or even require extra office visits. Sugar-rich foods can make hygiene harder and cause calculus build-up and cavities. You're probably already monitoring and limiting your child's intake of such foods, so there's really nothing new under the sun here. But, for the record, here are the "featured

2Prescription pain pills with dangerous side effects are not needed. Any orthodontist or dentist easily prescribing such drugs is not to be trusted. As you are no doubt aware from the news, opioid addiction is rampant. Pain drugs are, contrary to early assertions by their manufacturers, proving to be extremely addictive for many people after nominal and legitimate use. I can't emphasize enough—we practice truly pain-free orthodontics.

items" that should be avoided during orthodontic treatment and wearing of braces:

1. **Rock-hard foods**: ice (don't chew ice!), nuts, popcorn (has hard kernels inside), peanut brittle, rock candy, whole apples and carrots (unless softened by boiling or steaming them), corn on the cob, hard pretzels, bagels, hard rolls, hard taco shells.
2. **Extra-sticky foods**: Jolly Ranchers or Starbursts or similar candies, bubble gum, taffy, and sticky Cinnabon rolls.
3. **Very chewy foods**: pizza crust, beef jerky, gummy bears. Note: no chewing on pencils or pens.
4. **Super sugary foods and drinks**: soda pop with sugar, ice cream, most cookies, and cake. Yes, this is the worst of the forbidden foods. Some kids will give you a tough time. But there are sugar-free versions of all these kinds of foods, to be made, baked, or store-bought.

We will speak about this with your son or daughter and give them a printed list, but *you* will have to reinforce, monitor, and provide some substitute foods to prevent mutiny or months of sulking. Most kids get it, though. When they understand how short or long the number of weeks of wearing braces will turn out to be, how comfortable or uncomfortable wearing them is, how maintaining hygiene while wearing them is, and how their results are linked to them staying away from the short list of harmful foods, they are pretty responsible about it. Most parents who are initially really worried about this tell us later it wasn't the horror show they'd imagined.

Emergencies

Many "emergencies" actually aren't and can be easily and safely remedied at home.

If your family or son or daughter are away from home and, say, they chomp down on a piece of toffee and break a piece of their braces, there is *always* a remedy. You are *not* going to cut your vacation short and rush to the airport! Again, often a remedy provided by our instructions can meet the urgent need until everybody gets back home.

Sports

Speaking of injuries, the question of sports versus braces worries kids and parents alike. These days, kids are *very* active in organized and school sports, some starting one as another's season is ending. You know this; you are coordinating the schedules and working as their unpaid chauffeur.

Good news: for every sport and every level of play, there is either an inexpensive off-the-shelf mouth guard or a slightly costlier, custom-fit mouth guard to provide an extra, suitable level of dental protection and to protect the braces themselves. In some sports, additional face masks or other equipment normally treated as an option can be added and used during the time period of the orthodontic treatment. Ask us for guidance for your child and their sport(s). Some mouth guards even come with insurance against dental injury, covering financial costs.

By the way, there are collegiate and pro athletes—even NFL players—getting orthodontic treatment and even wearing braces. If they can, your child can! You do *not* need the drama of stopping your child from playing the sports they're committed to because of their orthodontic treatment.

See, this *isn't* going to be difficult!

Tips for Helping Your Child Adjust to a Life with Braces

- **All the cool kids are doing it (or soon will be):** Braces are a very popular appliance during the middle school and high school years. Rather than focus on how he or she feels wearing braces, encourage your child to begin actively looking for other kids who are wearing braces. Chances are, they'll find lots more than they ever imagined!
- **Even famous people do it:** Gwen Stefani. Prince Harry. Drew Barrymore. Tom Cruise. Dakota Fanning. Danny Glover. The list of famous people who've worn braces—many of them as adults—could fill half this book. Share with your child how even the most famous people in the spotlight sometimes need a little help through braces.
- **Forward thinking:** Yes, we do change lives—one smile at a time! By maintaining a long-term perspective, you can maintain motivation. It will be well worth the journey at the end when you obtain a smile you will enjoy the rest of your life!

Call us at **813-661-1073** or go to **TurkeOrthodontics.com** to schedule your own Customized Smile Analysis.

Chapter Nine

Life After Braces: Retainers

SO, YOUR CHILD'S BRACES are off and they're ready to live a life full of confidence and good oral health. They may think, *I'm free! I'm free!* Well, not quite yet.

The selection of the right braces, the expert orthodontist, and the compliant wearing of the braces gets us about three-fourths of the way to where we want to be: a well-aligned, as-perfect-as-possible, healthy smile for life.

But after braces, there are retainers.

While many patients are understandably eager to be done with braces once they come off, the fact is, retainers do as much work—if not more—than the braces themselves. Straight teeth in proper alignment have to stay that way, and for that, retainers are a big help.

When the braces are removed, teeth can still shift if not helped through a period of adjustment to settle in. Retainers gently but purposefully remind the teeth to stay straight during this adjustment period. It's advised that nearly all patients who've gone through the time, work, and expense of braces will want to use their removable retainers for life. Some dentists doing braces won't tell you this, but I will. Years ago, clinicians believed that once teeth were straightened by braces, they would simply stay that way forever. New science says otherwise. In fact, teeth position shifting as we age is to be expected. Teeth naturally shift to the middle and crowd. So, retainers are actually extremely important in maintaining the new smile from braces. Any claims otherwise, by some "brand" of braces or any doctor, are flat-out false.

Retainers can play a role in bruxism, which is the grinding of teeth when asleep. Wearing retainers at night can help protect your teeth from being worn down from this common night time habit.

Chapter Ten

Let's Celebrate!

HAVING TO WEAR BRACES can last for six months to two years or more in certain cases. During the time your child has them, they may have moved from child to preteen or preteen to teen, at times feeling embarrassed by having them, and possibly missing out on some things. They probably gave up favorite foods and snacks. They at least had to be super-conscious of what they ate and didn't eat. It's been a long time since they could sink their teeth into an apple!

You endured whatever complaining there was. You traded time to the office visits. You dealt with the "uh-oh!" and the "now what did you do?" emergencies if there were any. And, of course, you paid the bill.

We like to see our patients celebrate getting their braces off. There are so many ways your child can celebrate, everything from writing a journal about their experience to recording a video that shares their experience and shows their new look.

Here are a few options your child may want to consider:

- **Throw a party**. Throwing a "braces are off" party is a great way to celebrate. They can invite their friends over, put out the foods that they've been longing for, and they can enjoy showing off those new straight teeth. Their friends will love being able to take part in the celebration.
- **Plan a photo shoot**. Your child deserves to show the world their new beautiful smile! Plan a photo shoot, so they can be one-on-one with a photographer and put their best smile forward. They'll get some great shots and can show all their friends on social media their new look.
- **Chew some gum**. Your child might have wanted to have gum for the longest time. Although it's not the best habit, they can take an afternoon to chew some gum and feel guilt and worry free. Chew to your heart's content!
- **Go caramel**. Now is the time your child can sink their teeth into something like a caramel apple. No more avoiding the caramel and cutting the apple into bite-sized pieces. Nope, they can actually eat a full caramel apple, right off the stick! They can get one at the mall or a carnival or even make one themselves. Either way, they'll love being able to bite into that sticky gooey sweetness worry free!
- **Picnic in the park**. Weather permitting, a picnic in the park will make for a fun celebration. Take some of your child's favorite outdoor games, invite the friends, and have a cooler filled with icy drinks. On the grill, you can plan for things like corn on the cob that your child had to largely avoid while wearing their braces. It will make for a memorable afternoon!

- **Have a potluck dinner**. Have your child's friends and family each bring a dish people with braces have to take precaution with. This will give them the chance to learn a little more about what you went through, and it'll be fun to see what options they come up with. Ask each of the guests to write down a comment about your child with or without her braces. Your potluck will be filled with interesting dishes, laughs, and a good time!
- **Eat some healthy foods.** Eat foods like fresh whole carrots, apples, and celery (ants on a log)!
- **Relax**. What could be better than spending a couple of hours being pampered, or perhaps a round of golf or fishing out on the lake? Not much! Take your child out—celebrate them making it through their treatment. They'll walk out feeling and looking great!

Doing some of these things, such as chewing gum, may still not be good for your child's teeth or their body overall. But doing it on a special occasion, and not making a habit out of it, won't cause any harm.

Of course, nobody can celebrate unless we *started*. There really is no time like the present.

Call us at **813-661-1073** or go to **TurkeOrthodontics.com** to schedule your own Customized Smile Analysis.

Chapter Eleven

What About My Smile?

MOM, DAD, I'M NOT going to kid you: if braces and/or orthodontic treatment was advised when you were eight or ten or twelve and, for whatever reason, it didn't happen, and you now have misaligned teeth, periodontal problems because of them, a smile you often hide, and/or jaw/TMJ pain, it may *not* be an easy fix. It may *not* even be fixable with orthodontics or braces. But, often to the surprise of adults, braces—including invisible braces—can do a significant amount of good for people thirty, forty, or even fifty years old. You may still be able to go from an embarrassing smile you often hide to a beautiful smile you love! You'll also be able to enjoy better oral health. Many adults see years of age disappear from their faces!

The only way to know what the options are is with a complete, expert orthodontic exam.

While some offices may not actively seek adult patients, many will treat a lot of parents of patients, just like you, and a number of them come from referrals. You can arrange for your exam by speaking to any of the treatment coordinators at the office.

It's important to get your son or daughter the orthodontic care they need at the earliest time they are known to need it and for it to be the best care available. When that doesn't happen, it often comes around to really bother that person later in life!

Please don't ask them to hide their smile, because their new smile could change their life!

Call us at **813-661-1073** or go to **TurkeOrthodontics.com** to schedule your own Customized Smile Analysis.

"Dr. Turke has treated all three of our children. He is kind, caring, and the results were spectacular."

—PATRICK E.

FAQ

Here is a handy resource guide of frequently asked questions and orthodontic terminology, many of which are answered throughout the book.

What might happen if your child's mouth doesn't quite "fit"?

The fact is, the sooner you straighten your child's smile, the faster it will develop as it should: straight, clean, and healthy!

Are there any celebrities who've worn braces?

Many! Gwen Stefani, Prince Harry, Drew Barrymore, Tom Cruise, Dakota Fanning, Danny Glover, and more.

Will I be able to afford my child's braces?

Not only are most orthodontic procedures cheaper than ever, but insurance, payment plans, and a variety of other financing options make braces more affordable than they've ever been.

Is it really such a big deal if my child has crooked teeth?

Unfortunately, yes. Eroding, crooked, or unaligned smiles can take time to happen, but the time to act is now. Orthodontic irregularities don't just heal on their own or "go away" if you ignore them.

What are some of the warning signs that my child might need to go to the orthodontist?

There are many, but here are a few of the most common: early or late loss of teeth, protruding teeth, grinding or clenching of teeth, and speech difficulty.

What kind of "side effects" are caused by crooked teeth?

Some of the more frequent ones I see include headaches, toothaches, mouth breathing, chipped or worn down teeth, snoring, and drooling.

What makes an orthodontist more qualified than a dentist?

Orthodontists are *dental specialists* who have completed two to three years of additional education beyond dental school to learn the proper way to align teeth and jaws.

Why should I choose a specialist for my child's orthodontic care?

Unique treatment requirements and otherwise difficult bite problems are common, everyday scenarios for your orthodontist. In the interest of receiving the most efficient and effective orthodontic treatment possible, choose an orthodontic specialist.

How do I know if my doctor is an orthodontist?

Only orthodontists can belong to the American Association of Orthodontists (AAO).

Why is early treatment so important?

Age seven is the earliest time your orthodontist can determine future jaw and tooth alignment. That's because, at the age of seven, your child's upper and lower permanent front teeth are developing. These teeth set the stage for future jaw position and serious problems can develop if they come into the wrong position.

Is there such a thing as a child being too old for braces?

Actually, there is. Case in point: waiting to take your child to the orthodontist until they are twelve or thirteen can create more of an orthodontic challenge to correct their teeth than if we had started planing treatment for their unique case earlier. We will evaluate the best time for your child to start treatment when you come in for your complimentary consultation.

What if I don't believe in early orthodontics?

Well, you're entitled to your opinion, but this is like saying you don't believe in the sun. You can hide from it, pretend it's not there, or refuse to acknowledge it, but the simple fact remains. If you're not aware of the potential risks, you can get burnt.

Will my child actually need braces at seven?

Probably not. While I inform parents their child needs an initial exam at age seven, I also mention that most children *will not need braces until eleven to thirteen years of age.*

What is a crossbite?

When the upper and lower teeth grow at different rates, or even when the lower jaw grows disproportionately with the upper jaw, something known as a "crossbite" can occur.

Where should I start to look for treatment if I'm concerned about my child's jaw development?

If you suspect your child might have a crossbite or other issues, approach your family dentist and ask about orthodontics.

Why should I address a crossbite?

Crossbites can lead to pain, discomfort, and lack of confidence as your child begins to feel insecure or even ostracized because of this very treatable, very normal series of jaw and teeth developments.

What is Invisalign?

The Invisalign system is the virtually invisible way to straighten your teeth and achieve the dazzling smile you've always dreamed of. Using advanced 3-D computer-imaging technology, the orthodontist depicts your complete treatment plan, from the initial position of your teeth to the final desired position.

What are the primary benefits of Invisalign?

Like the word that inspired them, Invisalign aligners are practically clear and as close to "invisible" as one can get. No one may even notice you're wearing these virtually invisible braces, making Invisalign a seamless fit with your lifestyle and day-to-day interactions with others.

How do I get started with Invisalign?

It's simple: just make an appointment with your local orthodontist for an initial consultation. Most doctors will offer a free initial consultation to see if you are a good candidate for Invisalign.

How will Invisalign effectively move my teeth?

Aligners are the foundation for, and work in unison with, the Invisalign system. Like brackets and arch wires are to braces, Invisalign aligners move teeth by using the appropriate placement of controlled force on your child's teeth.

How many patients are being treated with Invisalign?

More than one million patients worldwide have been treated with Invisalign. The number of Invisalign smiles grows daily.

How does Invisalign Teen work?

Aligners snap on your teeth easily. They are comfortable and practically invisible. Invisalign Teen allows permanent teeth to grow and gently and continuously moves your teeth in small increments. Aligners are worn for about one to two weeks, then you swap them for a new pair.

Why are metal braces still so popular?

Metal braces are very strong and can withstand most types of treatment. Today's metal braces are smaller, sleeker, and more polished than ever before.

Are so-called "clear braces" effective?

Adults and teenagers like to choose ceramic braces because they "blend in" with the teeth and are less noticeable than metal. These are the types of braces actor Tom Cruise had.

Are clear braces appropriate for adults?

Absolutely! Adults of all ages can enjoy the same cosmetic and health benefits of properly aligned teeth.

What are some of my payment options in addition to insurance?

One way many patients pay for their procedures is by utilizing the benefits of what is known as "flex spending," where their employer matches their spending commitment.

Can a salt water rinse help deal with irritation caused by braces?

Absolutely; warm saltwater rinses soothe the cheek lining, which can get aggravated by your child's braces. Just remember to rinse and spit and don't swallow the salty water, or else your stomach will give you feedback!

How do I make a salt water rinse?

To make a salt water rinse, mix half a teaspoon of table salt in one cup of warm water. Stir until the salt is completely dissolved. Gently swish about a fourth of the cup in your mouth for thirty seconds. Make sure you force the water over the areas that feel sore. Then spit the water into the sink. Repeat until the entire cup is gone.

What if my child plays sports and needs a mouth guard?

The best advice for patients or parents looking for a mouth guard can be obtained from your pediatrician, dentist, pediatric dentist, orthodontist or oral surgeon. All of these specialists are uniquely trained to offer customized advice in order to help you prevent a sports-related dental or facial injury.

What about brushing with braces?

Here are some simple tips you can share with your child for the best results when brushing with braces on:

- Brush your teeth with a soft nylon toothbrush after each time you eat and before bed.
- Brush, rinse, and look; if you find any areas that are not clean, brush them again.
- Brush your gums as you brush your teeth (massage and stimulate).
- If no toothpaste is available, brush without.
- Floss your teeth once a day. The last time you eat or when you are ready for bed, you want to brush, rinse, floss, then rinse again.

- If you are unable to brush, rinse your mouth vigorously with water.
- Replace your old toothbrush when it gets worn out.
- It is absolutely essential that you continue regular visits to your family dentist for checkups and cleanings throughout your orthodontic treatment!

What type of foods should my child avoid while wearing braces?

There are four main types of food your child should avoid while wearing braces: (1) **hard foods**, like ice, popcorn, peanut brittle, rock candy, and corn on the cob, (2) **sticky foods**, like caramels, bubble gum, taffy, and suckers, (3) **chewy foods**, like pizza crust, crusty breads, beef jerky, and gummy bears, and (4) **sugary foods and drinks**, like cake, ice cream, cookies, pie, candy, and soda pop.

Why are retainers so important?

As we age, teeth naturally shift to the middle and crowd. Combined with late growth of the lower jaw, shifting of the teeth is expected following orthodontic treatment. Therefore, retainers are extremely important in the maintenance of your new smile following orthodontic treatment.

Resources

Before or after your consultation, you may want more information for yourself or your son or daughter. The following websites provide valuable insight to help you make the right decision for your child.

Braces.org is the "all about braces site" of the American Association of Orthodontists. This is the official regulatory body and professional association of orthodontists, and *only* orthodontists (*not* dentists) can be members. Here you will receive accurate, up-to-date information on orthodontics.

ExcellenceInOrthodontics.org is the elite association of orthodontists subscribing to a pledge of clinical and customer services excellence. A complete collection of information for patients and parents can be found here.

About the Author

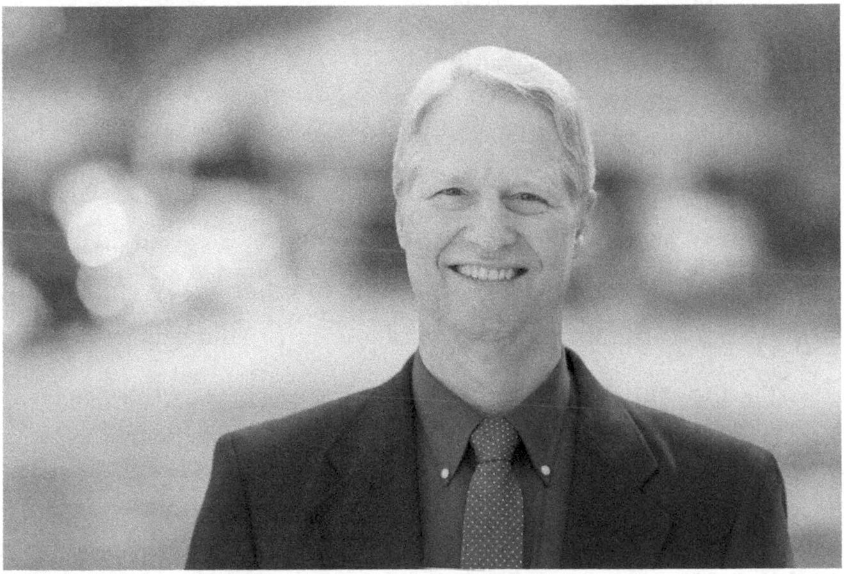

DR. ERIC TURKE is a speaker, teacher, author and orthodontic specialist. Dr. Turke is a faculty orthodontic instructor at the New York University Langone Dental Medicine Advanced Education in Pediatric Dental Residency Program located at the Suncoast Community Health Center in Brandon, Florida teaching other dental specialists about orthodontics. He maintains private practices in Brandon and Tampa, Florida. Dr. Turke completed his undergraduate studies at the University of South Florida in Tampa. He went on to receive his doctor of dental surgery degree with honors from New York University College of Dentistry.

He then completed his certificate of advanced graduate study in orthodontics and dentofacial orthopedics at New York University College of Dentistry.

Dr. Turke continues to study the latest advances in his specialty through memberships in the following professional organizations:

- American Association of Orthodontists
- American Dental Association
- Florida Dental Association
- Hillsborough County Dental Association

He has maintained active membership in the Christian Medical and Dental Society. Dr. Turke has also been involved in several medical and dental mission trips, both internationally and locally. The mission trips meet both physical and spiritual needs.

Dr. Eric Turke and his wife reside in Tampa, Florida and are the proud parents of three grown daughters.

What Motivated Me to be An Orthodontist That Changes Lives—One Smile at a Time

Helping people is part of my family culture. My dad was a physician and an OB/GYN. I admired the important work he did, but I also saw that his opportunities to spend time with his family were limited by the demands of his practice, and that didn't appeal to me; I wanted to be more of a family man, so I looked for a specialty in the medical field that would allow me to have more of a work/life balance.

During my studies at University of South Florida, I volunteered with and shadowed doctors in several different disciplines. I eventually approached the orthodontist at my church and asked for the opportunity to shadow him in his practice.

I'd never had braces myself, so it was a revelation to me. He became a mentor, letting me work with him in the office and in the lab. Working chairside, I saw how his work changed the lives of his patients by greatly improving their confidence to smile, how their orthodontic treatment improved their speech and also improved their ability to chew their food. I knew their treatment would enhance their self-confidence. What a great profession to be in, I thought, smiles really do change lives!

I went on to get my orthodontics degree at New York University years later, met and married my wife, and moved back to Tampa, Florida, where I opened my practice and got on with the job of changing lives, one smile at a time.

How Orthodontics Really Can Change Lives

In the twenty-five plus years that I've been in orthodontics, I've lost count of how many of my teenaged patients have told me how getting braces greatly enhanced their confidence and the social aspect of their lives; no more being bullied or being too timid to smile.

I think of the many times I've helped young, working professionals grow their confidence via orthodontic treatment to move into jobs that involved working with the public. Many of those patients would share with me that their parents did not have the funds to fix their smiles when they were younger, but their first investment as professionals was in braces—and they are uniformly glad they made that investment. Many single or newly single people came to me to get the smiles they'd always wanted, smiles that gave them the confidence they needed to re-enter the dating pool—and I'm glad to report that several of the ladies come in to show off their new engagement rings during the course of treatment.

Most adults have put off their own treatment for years, often because their childrens' needs seemed more pressing. I remember one lady in particular who was in her sixties when she came to see me about her smile and her bite; when we took her braces off at the end of treatment, she wrapped me in a bear hug and literally lifted me off the ground, saying, "Dr. Turke, I wanted to change my smile all my life and you did it!" It just goes to show that caring about how you look doesn't simply stop because you hit a particular age, nor should it.

Most of my practice is with children and teens, and many of them come in showing the unmistakable signs of having been bullied because of the appearance of their teeth. They don't smile, they tend to look down when speaking, and they cover their mouths if they laugh. But it's usually the mothers who tell me what's going on—"Susan's getting picked on at school and being called names." It's great to see the parents light up when I assure them that we can fix that.

Sometimes if the child is too young for full-blown treatment, we can do something simple just to alleviate the most obvious issues. Orthodontists think like firefighters: our first move is to rescue the patient from immediate distress, since kids who are being picked on aren't only socially isolated but are also likely to be falling behind their peers at school, because they just won't raise their hands or speak up in class.

I can tell you that years of research have served to prove what common sense tells us: people who have low self-esteem very often fail to reach their true potential whether that's in school, in terms of their career and earning capacity, or in more personal, social ways. Those who have gone through life hating their smiles are more apt to describe themselves as discontented with their lives. We can talk about the costs associated with orthodontics, but it honestly doesn't amount to much when you stack it up against a lifetime of feeling "less than" or unattractive. And as we all know, whether it's fair or not, we nearly all judge others by their appearance. That happens in the first seconds we meet someone, and in those first moments we make a lot of assumptions about the person we're meeting based on how they look. Are they smart? Educated? Leaders or followers? Attractive? Potential spouses? If your child's smile or your smile creates a bad first impression, it's awfully hard to turn that around.

Giving Back

Years ago, I was approached by friends of mine who had established a Christian missionary outreach with dentists, physicians and pharmacists, going to different third-world countries to help meet the physical and spiritual needs of the people there. They asked me to join them on a mission trip to Myanmar, a third-world country formerly known as Burma, where orthodontics and even basic dental care is quite rare. I accepted and, since then, have gone back several times. Our primary contact there is a Christian seminary. They reach out to their community through their churches. We set up our dental chairs and equipment in their churches, seminary, and schools to work on the local people and the seminary students as well. The townspeople will line up outside the door, and we examine them and determine what they need, in terms of medical and dental treatments, and do our best to provide it then and there. Also, several of the local churches support orphanages in the countryside in many different parts of the country, so we visit their orphanages and treat the children there. An orphanage here in the United States is a very different kind of place than one in a third-world country. Even those of us who have been on these trips before find it impossible not to tear up at the awful poverty and conditions these children live in. Yet they're so curious and friendly—like children anywhere—and so grateful for our help. They're precious; they come up to us and hug us—so grateful for the dental care they receive.

I've taken my children on various mission trips because I wanted them to be aware of the kind of need that exists in the world, and our individual responsibility to be a good steward of our talents.

Think That You or Your Child May Need Orthodontics? Please Don't Wait!

If you take nothing else from this book, I sincerely hope that one message will stick with you. If you think your child needs orthodontics or is likely to when they're older, don't wait to see an orthodontist. The difference between timely early treatment in situations where it's needed, and waiting, can mean less happy outcomes, longer and more complex treatment, and greater expense.

While the recommended age for that first orthodontic exam is seven, many parents put it off because they assume nothing can or should be done about a problem with their child's teeth until all the adult teeth are in place. That's wrong for a few reasons, and I'd like you to understand why.

First, you don't have to wait until your child's baby teeth are gone for me to be able to see any serious developmental problems that may be developing. If, for instance, your child has jaws that are too narrow to properly accommodate his adult teeth when they do come in, that's something we can see and treat early on much more easily than later. The reason for this is biological; your child's jawbones don't fuse until they're twelve or so, so before then, it's much easier to use an appliance called an expander to widen the jaw. Biology is on our side at that point, because the bone will fill in as it grows to accommodate the wider jaw. But if you wait, it can become much more challenging, because it's no longer so easy to widen the jaw. This can mean surgery down the line, whereas timely intervention would have been quicker and far less uncomfortable.

Another good reason to get in early is if your child is being picked on for her or his appearance. While we more than likely will not do extensive work on them at a young age, we can almost always do something that will make them look better and be less self-conscious, and save the more extensive work for down the line. Believe me, by the time you've read this book, you'll understand much better how important that intervention is, and the sooner the better.

It's also a good idea to let your child get to know the orthodontist and to see what it's all about. There's no charge for that initial exam and consultation, and you will leave with a much clearer idea of what, if anything, will be needed, and when. That helps you plan financially and personally in advance for treatment, and makes the whole process much easier to deal with when it really is time to get your child into braces.

Some people are suffering under the misconception that they need a referral from their dentist to come in, but that's not the case.

Whether or not you or your dentist thinks your child needs to see an orthodontist, my suggestion is that you go ahead and do it anyhow. There's no earthly reason not to, and you may save yourself and your child a whole lot of expense and discomfort down the road. And in many cases, an orthodontist will be able to spot problems a dentist doesn't have the training or equipment to catch.

Whether it's in my work here at home, in my own practice with the children and adults of our great community, or in the various places locally and across the world in which I'm blessed to use skills to help the less fortunate—I truly believe that smiles do change lives. The fact that you're reading this book tells me you're probably considering orthodontics for yourself or your child, and I hope you'll give me a call. We're here to answer any questions you might have, and would love the opportunity to greet you in our offices and show you around. I know you have choices—and I think that once you've met us and seen how we treat our patients, we'll be your first choice.

THE NEXT STEP

Your Customized Smile Analysis

When you are ready, I urge you to schedule your complimentary orthodontic evaluation at our office. We change smiles one person at a time! Yes, smiles change lives!

Call us at **813-661-1073** or go to **TurkeOrthodontics.com**.

Printed in the USA
CPSIA information can be obtained
at www.ICGtesting.com
JSHW012041140824
68134JS00033B/3193

9 781599 329420